DR. SEBI CURE FOR ALL DISEASES

The Ultimate Step-by-Step Guide on How to Effectively Cure Chronic Common Diseases and Detox the Liver in 9 Steps.

Table of Contents

Introduction

Sebi's name arose in the aftermath of the brutal and sad death of Nipsey Hussle (née Ermias Asghedom). On Sunday afternoon, March 31, the 33-year-old Los Angeles–based hip-hop musician and entrepreneur was brutally shot to death. Instead of focusing on his life and the nature of gun violence in America, we're now interested in a series of conspiracy theories about why Hussle was slain.

Hussle's premature death On Sunday afternoon (March 31st), the Los Angeles rapper had just acquired the plaza where his Marathon Clothing business was located. According to a Forbes article about Hussle's entrepreneurship, Hussle intended to rebuild the area as a six-story residential building atop a commercial plaza, along with a new iteration of his clothing store, in the hopes of "giving opportunities and jobs to all communities and improving the neighborhood."

Hussle was also working on a documentary on Alfredo Bowman, better known as the late Dr. Sebi, an unlicensed physician who claimed in the late 1980s that he could treat AIDS.

"I'm working on a documentary about the trial in 1985...when Dr. Sebi went to trial against New York because he stated in the papers that he treated AIDS," Hussle said in a 2018 Breakfast Club interview that leaked shortly after his death. "He won the lawsuit, then the next day he won the case in federal court...the tale is significant."

"If I could say, 'Hey, somebody cured AIDS,' you'd be like, 'Yeah, right,'" he added. "And then I could show you an example of him going to trial and demonstrating in court to a jury that he healed AIDS, and you'd be interested in that."

In a previous interview, Hussle discussed the documentary with novelist and documentarian Tariq Nasheed and even joked that the project may lead to his death.

Some doubters, however, think that the rapper's death was an attempt by the American government and pharmaceutical industry to suppress the late Bowman's work.

This is not a coincidence! Nipsey Hussle was working on a documentary on Dr. Sebi's trial in 1985. Dr. Sebi claimed that he could cure AIDS and was reportedly killed by U.S. Medical Corporations because his AIDS treatment would reduce their revenues.

Bowman died in Honduras in 2016 as a result of respiratory problems that developed while he was in prison on money laundering allegations. But, before his death, he had built a name for himself in the United States as a herbalist and holistic doctor.

Bowman's life is poorly recorded and unknown. His website offers a brief description of his upbringing in Honduras with his grandmother, who first exposed him to herbal treatment, and his migration to the United States, where he was diagnosed with "asthma, diabetes, impotency, and obesity."

"After fruitless treatments with conventional doctors and traditional western medicine, Sebi was led to a herbalist in Mexico," where he achieved "great healing results from all his ailments," according to the report. Bowman was inspired by his personal healing experience to "begin developing natural plant cell food components aimed towards inter-cellular cleaning and the rejuvenation of all the cells that comprise the human body."

He subsequently shared the compounds with others, which led to the establishment of the USHA Research Institute (in Brooklyn, New York), Dr. Sebi LLC, and the USHA Healing Village (USHA) in La Ceiba, Honduras. Bowman created a number of goods via these businesses, including "Cell Prolifirant Eva-Therapeutic Salve," "Hair Food," "Horadin," "Limphaslin," "Nervino," "Sperma I," "Testee II," and "Uturin."

Bowman was even offering a $1,500 "All-Inclusive" package that promised to cleanse "the body on the molecular level by breaking down acid, mucus, poisons, and calcifications."

By the 1980s, Bowman was selling his goods in the United States while still practicing medicine through his Brooklyn-based institute. Bowman was charged with two charges of practicing medicine without a license in 1987 and brought to court by Robert Abrams, the New York Attorney General at the time. The charge arose from advertising he posted in the Village Voice and the Amsterdam News telling people they might be cured of AIDS, herpes, leukemia, lupus, sickle cell anemia, and other illnesses for a $500 initial cost and $80 for each successive appointment. Bowman's USHA also claimed to have "cured" AIDS.

The trial ended in a significant judgment in Brooklyn Supreme Court, when the jury ruled Bowman not guilty of the charges. Two undercover operatives were connected with a tiny audio recorder and dispatched to Bowman's institution to "entrap Sebi into giving a medical diagnosis." The tape recording, however, "failed to convince the jury that Sebi did, in fact, give a medical diagnosis," according to a New Amsterdam research on the trial.

"What was noteworthy about the verdict is that USHA's African Bio-Mineral Balance will now be recognized across the world," Simeon Greenaway, Bowman's attorney, stated at the time. (The African Bio-Mineral Balance was a "therapeutic strategy" that benefitted "the nutritional demands of the African gene structure.")

However, there was a successful legal lawsuit against USHA in which the firm agreed not to make therapeutic claims for any of its products.

The agreement prohibited "Ogun Herbal Research Institute (d/b/a USHA), Fig Tree Products Company, and their principals, officers, directors, employees, agents, successors, heirs, and assigns, as well as Alfredo Bowman and Maa Bowman, their successors, heirs, and assigns" from "claiming, orally or in writing, directly or by implication, that respondents, their services, or their products can cure, mitigate, or in.

"When I informed my mother I had treated my twelfth AIDS patient; she said, 'They are going to get you,'" Bowman claimed in a 2015 appearance on The Rock Newman Show, where he claims to have defended himself. "... The judge stated I had to present one of each patient I had treated... "I choose 77."

Bowman also explained how he cured his AIDS patients in the interview, saying he helped someone named Michael White in Boston by producing a chemical "made to cleanse the cells."

Bowman stated, "I removed lactose, uric acid, and carbonic acid from the man's diet." "Milk, carbohydrates, and meat. He began to heal in 24 hours after eliminating these foods from his diet and then cleaning his cells."

Following the case, the USHA Research Institute and Bowman relocated to California, where he expanded his clientele to include celebrities such as Lisa "Left Eye" Lopes (the late TLC artist had visited Bowman in Honduras prior to her death), Steven Seagal, John Travolta, Eddie Murphy, and Michael Jackson, whom Bowman claimed to have cured of his painkiller addiction.

According to The Telegraph's obituary for Bowman, "In June 2004, Jackson was said to be spending $3,960 a night at Loews Miami Beach Hotel meditating and praying with Sebi (described as a "witch doctor" in some sources) to prepare for his impending trial on nine allegations of child abuse."

Later that year, Bowman sued Jackson for $380,00 in unpaid invoices after the late pop icon's brother Randy gave him $10,000 as "payment in full" for his services. The case was dropped in 2015 due to a lack of prosecution.

Bowman was detained and charged with money laundering by the Honduran government in 2016 after attempting to move from a commercial flight from the United States to a private jet at an airport in Honduras. According to prior accounts, Bowman was traveling with $37,000 in cash and was freed awaiting a court hearing, only to be detained again on June 3 by the Ministerio Publico — Honduras' version of the FBI — and accused of money laundering. Bowman's family sought to gain his release and claimed that he got pneumonia while in prison but were unsuccessful. Bowman died on August 6, 2016, at the age of 82.

A conspiracy theory concerning Hussle's killing grew out of a conspiracy theory about Bowman's death. Supporters think that the lack of public attention to not just his death but also his triumph in court has silenced his legacy, arguing that he was a threat to the pharmaceutical business. Others, on the other hand, see Bowman as a pseudoscientist and propagator of erroneous Afrocentric ideas, whose approach to dealing with illnesses like AIDS diminishes the seriousness of the disease.

1

Cleansing and Detoxification: Key to Reversing Disease

Detoxification, often known as detox, is a trendy term. It generally refers to following a certain diet or using specific products that claim to rid your body of toxins, thus improving your health and helping weight loss.

Fortunately, your body is able to eliminate toxins without the need for specific diets or expensive supplements.

However, you can assist your body's natural detoxification process.

Complete body detox is a procedure that some individuals believe might help the body remove toxins. It might entail following a certain diet, fasting, taking supplements, or utilizing a sauna.

Detoxes can stimulate behaviors that can help the body's natural detoxification processes, such as eating a healthy diet, exercising regularly, and staying hydrated.

There are, however, dangers involved, and certain detox products might be hazardous.

What does a full body detox involve?

A complete body detox, often known as a cleanse, is a regimen that people follow in order to remove toxins from their bodies.

Toxins, often known as poisons or pollutants, are chemicals that have a detrimental impact on health. These chemicals can already be eliminated by the body on its own via the liver, kidneys, digestive system, and skin.

Detox proponents say that detox can aid in this process. There is no one definition of what a complete body detox entails, although it may need that a person:

- Follow a specific diet
- Use colonic irrigation, enemas, or laxatives
- Use a sauna
- Reduce exposure to toxins in their environment
- Fast
- Drink more water or juices
- Use supplements

Are they necessary?
While some people feel that full body detoxes are beneficial to their health, they are not essential for the majority of people. Toxins are already eliminated from the body by the body's own very effective detoxification mechanism.

Sometimes people have medical problems that necessitate detoxification assistance. Chelation treatment, for example, may be used to treat heavy metal toxicity. This is a method of removing heavy metals from the body.

People who are in good health, on the other hand, rarely require further detoxification assistance.

Potential Benefits
While detoxes are not medically essential for the majority of individuals, they may provide some health advantages in specific instances, such as:

Weight loss: According to 2017 research, detoxification diets can result in weight reduction. The researchers do caution, however, that this is most likely owing to the extreme calorie restriction of some regimens.

Fruits and vegetables: Many detox diets include the consumption of fruits and vegetables. Nearly three-quarters of Americans, according to the Office of Disease Prevention and Health Promotion, do not consume enough fruits and vegetables.

Hydration: Many full body detoxes encourage water consumption as well. Water is essential for good health because it helps the body eliminate waste through perspiration, urine, and bowel movements.

Antioxidants: According to a 2014 study, several research has discovered that some detox diets might help with liver function and that specific food can boost the antioxidant glutathione. Toxins such as heavy metals can be removed from the body with the aid of glutathione. However, the researchers point out that many of these studies had problems in their design, either had a limited number of participants or were animal studies.

Many of the possible advantages of detoxes are short-lived and disappear once a person returns to their regular diet. At the moment, the evidence does not support the use of detox diets for weight loss or toxin removal.

Potential Risks

According to the National Center for Complementary and Integrative Health, some detoxes are harmful to people's health because they encourage them to:

- Reduce food consumption, resulting in a shortage of essential nutrients.

- Drinking excessive amounts of juices or teas might result in a hazardous electrolyte imbalance.
- Drink juices high in oxalates, which may increase your risk of renal issues.
- Use detox solutions, including laxatives, to avoid severe diarrhea and dehydration.
- Experiment with diet regimens that aggravate underlying illnesses such as diabetes.

Because some detox products include dangerous or unlawful chemicals, the Food and Drug Administration (FDA) and the Federal Trade Commission (FTC) have taken action against firms marketing them.

Before attempting supplements, detox products, or new diets, people should always consult with a doctor or a nutritionist.

Common Misconceptions about Detoxing

Detox diets are believed to rid your body of toxins, enhance your health, and encourage weight reduction. They frequently include the use of laxatives, diuretics, vitamins, minerals, teas, and other detoxifying foods.

The term "toxin" is used loosely in the context of detox diets. Pollutants, synthetic chemicals, heavy metals, and processed foods are all prevalent, and all have negative health effects. Popular detox diets, on the other hand, seldom reveal the toxins they're trying to get rid of or how they're doing it.

Furthermore, there is no evidence that these diets are effective for toxin removal or long-term weight reduction. Toxins are eliminated by the body through a complex process, including the liver, kidneys, digestive system, skin, and lungs.

However, only when these organs are in good health are they able to properly remove undesirable chemicals.

So, while detox diets don't accomplish anything your body can't do on its own, they can help you maximize your body's natural cleansing mechanism. While detox diets seem appealing, your body is perfectly capable of dealing with toxins and other undesirable things.

Nine ways to rejuvenate your body's detoxification system on the base of evidence.

1. Limit alcohol.

More than 90% of alcohol is processed in the liver. Alcohol is metabolized by liver enzymes to acetaldehyde, a recognized carcinogen. When your liver recognizes acetaldehyde as a toxin, it changes it to a harmless molecule called acetate, which is then removed from your body.

While observational studies have indicated that low-to-moderate alcohol intake is good for heart health, excessive drinking can lead to a slew of health issues. Excessive alcohol use can harm your liver function by generating fat accumulation, inflammation, and scarring.

When this happens, your liver is unable to operate properly and fulfill its essential functions, such as filtering waste and other toxins from your body.

As a consequence, limiting or abstaining from alcohol is one of the most effective ways to keep your body's detoxification system running properly.

According to health authorities, ladies should have one drink per day and males should consume two drinks per day. For the potential cardiac benefits of light-to-moderate drinking, if you don't drink today, you shouldn't start. Too much alcohol decreases your liver's capacity to perform its regular tasks, such as detoxification.

2. Focus on sleep.

A good night's sleep is essential for supporting your body's health and natural detoxifying mechanism. Sleeping helps your brain to restructure and rejuvenate itself while also removing harmful waste byproducts that have been collected over the day.

One of these waste products is beta-amyloid, a protein that leads to the development of Alzheimer's disease. When you don't get enough sleep, your body doesn't have enough time to complete those processes, so toxins build up and negatively affect your health.

In the short and long term, stress, anxiety, high blood pressure, heart disease, type 2 diabetes, and obesity have all been linked to a lack of sleep.

To maintain excellent health, you should sleep seven to nine hours every night on a regular basis. If you have trouble remaining or falling asleep at night, making lifestyle adjustments such as adhering to a sleep routine and reducing blue light generated by mobile devices and computer screens before going to bed might help. Adequate sleep helps your brain to restructure, rejuvenate, and remove toxins that build up during the day.

3. Drink more water.

Water does a lot more than just satisfy your thirst. It keeps your body temperature stable, lubricates joints, promotes digestion and nutrition absorption, and detoxifies your body by eliminating waste materials.

Your body's cells must be repaired on a regular basis in order to function correctly and break down nutrients for your body to use as energy.

However, these activities produce wastes in the form of urea and carbon dioxide, which may be harmful if they accumulate in your blood.

Water transports these wastes, which are effectively eliminated via urine, breathing, or perspiration. As a consequence, it's essential to remain hydrated throughout detoxification. Men should drink 125 ounces (3.7 liters) of water per day, while women should drink 91 ounces (2.7 liters).

You may need more or less depending on your diet, where you live, and how much activity you do. Water, in addition to its various functions in your body, assists your body's detoxification system in removing waste materials from your blood.

4. Reduce your intake of sugar and processed foods.

Sugar and processed meals are believed to be the underlying causes of today's public health issues. Obesity and other chronic illnesses such as heart disease, cancer, and diabetes have been related to a high intake of sugary and highly processed meals.

These illnesses impair your body's capacity to cleanse itself naturally by damaging vital organs such as your liver and kidneys. Excessive use of sugary drinks, for example, may lead to fatty liver, a condition that affects liver function.

By consuming less junk food, you can keep your body's detoxification system healthy.
You may restrict your intake of junk food by leaving it on the store shelf. The absence of it in your kitchen eliminates the temptation entirely.

Replacing junk food with healthier options such as fruits and vegetables is another good strategy to cut back on intake.
Obesity and diabetes have been related to excessive junk food intake. These diseases can damage organs involved in detoxification, such as your liver and kidneys.

5. Eat antioxidant rich foods.

Antioxidants help to protect your cells from free radical damage. which are substances. An excessive amount of free radicals causes oxidative stress. Your body produces these substances naturally for cellular functions including digestion. Alcohol, cigarette smoking, a poor diet, and pollution exposure, on the other hand, may generate an excessive amount of free radicals.

These chemicals have been linked to a variety of diseases, including dementia, heart disease, liver disease, asthma, and some forms of cancer, by causing harm to your body's cells. Eating an antioxidant-rich diet can help your body battle oxidative stress, which is produced by excess free radicals and other pollutants that raise your risk of illness.

Concentrate on acquiring antioxidants through food rather than pills, which may actually raise your risk of some diseases if consumed in excessive quantities. Antioxidants include vitamins A, C, and E, as well as selenium, lycopene, lutein, and zeaxanthin. Berries, fruits, nuts, chocolate, vegetables, spices, and drinks such as coffee and green tea contain high levels of antioxidants.

A diet high in antioxidants helps your body minimize free radical damage and may lessen your risk of illnesses that interfere with detoxification.

6. Eat foods high in prebiotics.

Gut health is essential for keeping your detoxification system healthy. A detoxification and excretion process in your intestinal cells protects your stomach and body from potentially harmful substances like toxins.

Prebiotics, a kind of fiber that feeds the good bacteria in your gut known as probiotics, are essential for good gut health. Prebiotics enable your good bacteria to generate nutrients known as short-chain fatty acids, which are helpful to your health.

Because of antibiotic usage, poor dental cleanliness, and poor food quality, the beneficial bacteria in your stomach might become imbalanced with harmful bacteria.

As a result, this unfavorable change in microorganisms might compromise your immunological and detoxification systems, increasing your risk of illness and inflammation.

Eating prebiotic-rich foods can help your immune and detoxification systems stay healthy. Prebiotic foods include tomatoes, artichokes, bananas, asparagus, onions, garlic, and oats.

Eating a prebiotic-rich diet helps to keep your digestive system healthy, which is essential for optimal detoxification and immunological function.

7. Decrease your salt intake.

Detoxing is a method for some people to get rid of extra water. Consuming too much salt can cause your body to retain extra fluid, especially if you have a kidney or liver disease or if you don't drink enough water.

This additional fluid accumulation may cause bloating and garment discomfort. You may cleanse your body of extra water weight if you consume an excessive quantity of salt.

While it may seem counterintuitive, increasing your water intake is one of the most effective ways to reduce water weight caused by too much salt.

This is due to the fact that when you ingest too much salt and not enough water, your body produces an antidiuretic hormone, which keeps you from urinating — and therefore detoxifying.

By increasing your water intake, your body decreases the release of the antidiuretic hormone and increases urination, allowing you to eliminate more water and waste. Increasing your consumption of potassium-rich foods, which counteracts some of the effects of salt, is also beneficial. Potassium-rich foods include potatoes, squash, kidney beans, bananas, and spinach.

Excessive salt consumption might cause water retention. Increase your consumption of water and potassium-rich meals to remove extra water — and waste.

8. Get active.

Regular exercise, regardless of body weight, has been linked to a longer life and a lower risk of a variety of illnesses and diseases, including type 2 diabetes, heart disease, high blood pressure, and some malignancies.

While there are numerous processes behind the health advantages of exercise, one of the most important is decreased inflammation. While some inflammation is required for infection recovery or wound healing, excessive inflammation weakens your body's systems and causes illness.

Exercise can assist your body's systems, particularly its detoxification system, work correctly and protect against disease by decreasing inflammation. It is suggested that you engage in at least 150–300 minutes of moderate-intensity exercise per week, such as brisk walking, or 75–150 minutes of vigorous-intensity physical activity per week, such as jogging.

Physical exercise on a regular basis reduces inflammation and helps your body's detoxification mechanism to function correctly.

9. Other helpful detox tips.

Despite the fact that there is no current evidence to support the efficacy of detox diets for removing toxins from the body, some dietary and lifestyle modifications may assist in lowering toxin load and boosting your body's detoxification mechanism.

Consume sulfur-containing foods. Sulfur-rich foods, such as onions, broccoli, and garlic, increase the excretion of heavy metals such as cadmium.

Take a look at chlorella. According to animal research, chlorella is a kind of algae that has various nutritional advantages and may aid in the removal of pollutants such as heavy metals.

Use cilantro to season meals. Cilantro aids in the elimination of some poisons, such as heavy metals like lead and chemicals like phthalates and pesticides.

Glutathione needs to be boosted. Sulfur-rich foods like eggs, broccoli, and garlic help to improve the function of glutathione, a major antioxidant produced by the body and involved in detoxification.

Use natural cleaning agents instead. Using natural cleaning solutions such as vinegar and baking soda instead of commercial cleaning agents can help to limit your exposure to potentially harmful chemicals.

Select natural body care. Natural deodorants, cosmetics, moisturizers, shampoos, and other personal care items can also help to decrease your chemical exposure.

Although promising, many of these benefits have only been demonstrated in animal research. As a consequence, human studies are needed to back up these findings. Some dietary and lifestyle modifications may aid your body's natural detoxification process.

2

How to Detox The Liver

Liver cleanses claim to clear the body of toxins and impurities, but their usage is contentious due to a lack of scientific evidence.

Products claiming to cleanse the liver may even be hazardous, and the Food and Drug Administration (FDA) in the United States does not regulate them. In this post, we'll look at how liver cleanses are said to work and what evidence there is to back them up.

What is liver cleanse?

The liver is the body's natural detoxifier, cleansing it of toxins and producing bile to aid with digestion. A healthy liver can cleanse nearly everything that a person comes into contact with. The liver is situated on the body's right side. immediately behind the rib cage. When the liver is damaged, the body's ability to filter out harmful chemicals is reduced.

This can result in a variety of symptoms, including:
- Gallstones
- Fatigue
- Nausea
- Diarrhea
- Itching
- Yellow jaundiced skin
- Swelling

- Blood vessel problems

Toxins are said to build in the liver throughout the filtration process, according to a number of natural health practitioners, supplement businesses, and medical websites. They claim that over time, these poisons can induce a variety of nonspecific symptoms, as well as severe illnesses or raise the risk of cancer. There is minimal evidence to back this up.

Chemical exposure, on the other hand, can cause liver damage over time. Drinking alcohol, for example, is a well-known strategy to degrade liver function over time.

A liver detox usually entails one or more of the following:
- Using supplements intended to remove toxins from the liver
- Eating a liver-friendly diet
- Avoiding certain foods
- Going on a juice fast
- Enemas are a kind of colon and intestinal cleanser.

While liver failure is a severe health issue, there is little evidence that hazardous poisons accumulate in normally healthy livers without particular exposure to high concentrations of these substances. Mainstream medical practitioners say that detoxifying the liver is unnecessary and possibly harmful.

Is it possible to lose weight by cleaning your liver?
Some liver cleanses claim to help people lose weight by boosting their metabolism. Supporters think that draining toxins from the liver might enhance metabolism. However, there is no data to back this up.

In reality, extremely low-calorie diets might cause the body's metabolism to decrease. This is due to the body's adaptation to reduced nutritional intake, which causes nutrients to be absorbed more slowly.

Some diets that promise to promote liver health require patients to eat very few calories over a period of several days. This might result in short-term weight reduction. The majority of the weight loss, however, is water weight, which will return as a person resumes regular eating habits.

Liver-friendly foods

While it is not feasible to cleanse the liver with any single meal or a mix of foods, physicians may advise patients with liver disease to make dietary modifications. Most people can lower their risk of liver disease by avoiding highly fatty meals and alcohol.

Doctors may provide the following dietary advice to patients suffering from particular liver diseases:

Bile duct disease: When cooking, use fat alternatives and kernel oil because the body requires less bile to break it down.

Cirrhosis: Limit your salt consumption. Protein intake may also need to be reduced, but only under the guidance of a doctor.

Fatty liver disease: Consume high-fiber meals while avoiding high-calorie foods.

Hemochromatosis: Iron-rich meals and iron supplements should be avoided. Consume no raw shellfish.

Hepatitis C: Iron-rich meals and iron supplements should be avoided. Reduce your salt consumption.

Wilson disease: Copper-rich foods, such as mushrooms, chocolate, and nuts, should be avoided. People with healthy livers don't need to follow any special diets. Simply eating a well-balanced, diverse diet and avoiding alcohol use can assist in protecting liver health.

Detoxing Your Liver: Fact Versus Fiction

Your liver is the major filtering system of the human body, turning pollutants into waste products, cleansing your blood, and metabolizing nutrients and medicines to supply the body with some of its most vital proteins. Because the liver is such an important element of the body's general control, it's critical to keep it healthy and avoid overindulgence.

Many products have entered the market in recent years claiming to detox and cleanse your liver, whether it's after a weekend of bingeing on food or alcohol, to maintain everyday liver function, or to heal an already damaged liver. Tinsay Woreta, M.D., a hepatologist at Johns Hopkins, is here to dispel recurring liver health misconceptions and assess the effectiveness of cleanses.

Myth #1: Liver cleanses are essential for everyday health maintenance and is especially beneficial after overindulging.

Though liver cleanses are marketed as a panacea for everyday liver health and overindulgence, Johns Hopkins hepatologists do not advocate them. "Unfortunately, because these products are not regulated by the FDA, they are not consistent and have not been thoroughly evaluated in clinical trials," says the author.

While certain popular liver cleanse components have been proven to be beneficial — milk thistle has been shown to decrease liver inflammation, and turmeric extract has been shown to protect against liver damage — others have not. — there is insufficient clinical trial data in humans to recommend routine use of these natural compounds for prevention.

When it comes to excessive alcohol or food intake, less is always better when it comes to liver health, and cleanses have not been proved to cure your body of the harm caused by excessive use.

Myth #2: Liver cleanses a good and safe approach to reducing weight.
Many liver detox treatments are also marketed as weight loss cleanses. However, there is no clinical evidence to back up the efficacy of these cleanses. In fact, certain nutritional supplements can actually injure the liver by causing drug-induced toxicity. Thus, they should be taken with caution.

Myth #3: You cannot prevent yourself from liver illness.
"Contrary to popular belief, there are several preventive measures you may take to protect yourself from liver disease," adds Woreta.

The following measures are suggested:
- **Do not drink alcohol in excess.** To avoid the development of alcoholic liver disease, males should not drink more than three drinks per day, and women should not drink more than two drinks per day on a regular basis.
- **Avoid weight gain.** Maintain a healthy body mass index (18 to 25) by eating well and exercising on a regular basis to reduce your chance of getting non-alcoholic fatty liver disease.
- **Beware of engaging in risky behaviors.** To reduce your chances of contracting viral hepatitis, avoid engaging in risky activities such as illegal drug use or unprotected intercourse with many partners.

- **Know your risk factors.** You should be tested if you have any of the following risk factors for liver disease, since chronic liver disease may lie undiagnosed for years:
  - Excessive alcohol use
  - Family history of liver disease

If you have any of the following hepatitis C risk factors, it's important to talk to your doctor about being tested, since almost half of the population is unaware they're infected:

- Anyone who had a blood transfusion before 1992
- Current or former illicit drug use
- Patients on hemodialysis
- Patients with HIV
- Health-care professionals who have been stabbed with needles containing hepatitis C-infected blood
- Anyone who has had tattoos done in an uncontrolled setting in the past.

Myth #4: The liver might help to repair any existing liver damage.

"Liver cleanses have not been shown to heal existing liver damage," adds Woreta, "but for individuals who are impacted, there are many alternative types of treatment available."

Here are a few examples of liver diseases and associated treatment options:

Hepatitis A and B are contagious. If you are not immune to hepatitis A or B, or if you have any other kind of liver illness, you should be vaccinated. There are also highly effective oral medicines available for people with chronic hepatitis B infection.

Alcoholism causes liver damage. To improve the liver's chances of mending, all alcohol use should be stopped. Once active damage has been halted, the liver has an incredible capacity to repair and recover.

Hepatitis C is a viral illness of the liver. Very effective treatment for hepatitis C well-tolerated oral medicines are now available.

Fatty liver disease is not caused by alcohol. Weight loss is the most effective treatment for the non-alcoholic fatty liver disease since it has been found to reduce the quantity of fat in the liver as well as the inflammation induced by the fat.

Myth #5: Obesity does not enhance your chances of developing liver disease.

Obesity raises your chances of having non-alcoholic fatty liver disease substantially. Fat in the liver, as described in Myth #4, can induce inflammation, which can contribute to the development of fibrosis and cirrhosis. "Because of the expanding obesity pandemic in the United States, the incidence of non-alcoholic fatty liver disease is quickly increasing and is anticipated to replace hepatitis C as the primary reason for liver transplantation over the next 30 years," adds Woreta.

Finally, the best thing you can do for your liver is to take good care of it. Avoid regular overconsumption of food and alcohol, follow a balanced diet and exercise routine, and be tested if you have risk factors for liver disease. If you do have liver impairment, consult with your doctor to devise the healthiest and safest treatment strategy for your specific requirements.

Simple Liver Detox Methods

The liver may not be the body's CEO, but it does have a seat in one of the corner offices.

The liver has two titles (organ, gland) and over 500 responsibilities to play on a daily basis for an organ that measures only two to four inches and weighs only two to three pounds. The liver, being the second biggest organ (after the skin), bears several significant duties that cannot be delegated.

In addition, the liver is the only organ that can lose up to 75% of its mass and yet regenerate to full size!

While most people are aware that excessive alcohol use may harm the liver, this is far from the only way the liver can be harmed. When the liver is injured or weakened, it is unable to fulfill its duty of detoxifying the body as effectively.

When this happens, the liver needs assistance. These easy liver detox methods can help your liver get back on its feet so it can accomplish its job of keeping you healthy.

Always with your doctor before changing your daily diet or health regimen if you are under a doctor's supervision for the treatment of any health concerns or are taking any needed drugs.

Drink plenty of water.

Simple liver detox treatments might appear, well, simple. But, in this case, the plain reality is that water aids the liver in moving toxins via its own cellular processes and speeding them out of your body.

However, not just any water will suffice to provide the full detoxifying benefit. At regular intervals throughout the day, drink filtered tap water at room temperature (aka., upon awakening, in between meals, early evening; not while eating and not too much 2 hours before bed). To boost its efficacy, add a sprinkle of salt and the spice turmeric to your water.

Aim for 4 liters of water each day as a basic rule of thumb. Avoid carbonated water and water in plastic beverage containers.

Sweat, sweat, and more sweat.

Depending on where you reside, you may be able to do this just by going for a stroll outside! However, this is not the best way to employ sweat as a liver cleanse. Exercise-induced perspiration has its own cleansing advantages, forcing toxins up from couch potatoes' comfortable chairs and transporting them out of the body with the sweat.

Toxins can be eliminated by hot yoga, a pleasant jog, HIT exercises, or a sauna session. Simply wipe away perspiration as quickly as possible with a toxin to prevent reabsorption of toxin back into the body, and take a cool shower immediately after sweating.

Don't scrimp on the shuteye.

Science is now beginning to grasp why humans require at least eight hours of uninterrupted sleep every night. Sleep is a detoxifier! Sleep is essential for regulating metabolism as well as targeting and removing brain and neurological toxins from the liver.

Sleep disables non-essential bodily activities, allowing the body to allocate its energy resources to digesting, repairing, restoring, and detoxifying.

The lymphatic system is a bodily system that works with the liver as you sleep to remove toxins while also repairing cognitive, physical, and behavioral functions that enhance mood, attention, and endurance.

Opt for anti-inflammatory meals.

Certain foods are inherently beneficial to liver function. Learning about these meals and incorporating them into a regular daily routine will help the liver accomplish its finest function.

As an added bonus, consuming foods with natural anti-inflammatory properties helps lower the risk of fatty liver disease, which occurs when the liver accumulates an abnormally large amount of fat.

Fatty liver disease, if left untreated, can progress to cirrhosis, a condition that causes persistent scarring and inhibits liver regeneration.

The good news is that a liver-healthy diet will also naturally support weight reduction or maintenance, more energy, better sleep, and a more youthful appearance.

All foods cultivated above ground, such as green vegetables, beans, grains, and mushrooms, have inherent anti-inflammatory qualities. These plant-based meals produce direct photosynthesis, which produces water, oxygen, and nutrients on which cells rely to operate properly. GMO crops wheat, corn, soy, alfalfa, canola, and items heavily sprayed with the dangerous pesticide Roundup (i.e., dairy products, eggs, poultry, red meat, pork, fish, sweet potatoes, potatoes, beets, sugar cane, coffee, nuts) are an exception because they are extremely harmful to the liver at any level of consumption.

Toxins should be reduced or eliminated from your regular activity.

This is the phase of the liver cleansing regimen that no one looks forward to. However, the plain reality is that the more poisons put into the bodily system, the more toxins the liver has to remove.

Adding to the liver's workload is never a good formula for a successful liver detox! Reducing or eliminating all animal protein, alcohol, sugar, wheat, maize, soy, nicotine, processed foods, caffeine, and nuts will provide your liver with much-needed rest and allow it to conduct some much-needed house cleaning.

Give the digestive system some assistance.

The more efficient your digestive system is in removing toxins, the less work it will pass on to the liver. Probiotics are one of the most beneficial digestive aids available. These small helpful bacteria get immediately to work, changing the power balance in the gut away from dangerous bacteria and toward healthy flora and fauna.

Probiotics can be found in fermented foods such as tiny beans boiled for three days, sauerkraut, kimchi, and pickles. Consume in tiny doses only once each day. Fermented foods like kombucha, miso, and kefir should be eaten in moderation since they can easily overburden the liver function, especially if it is already impaired.

Many people are first apprehensive or resistant to attempting a liver detox since the entire procedure appears new and even complex. However, as these six suggestions demonstrate, it is actually extremely simple to assist the liver in its detoxification!

Plus, there are so many other advantages to incorporating these six easy techniques into daily life that it almost seems like a no-brainer to give them a shot.

Other methods for improving liver health

Some easy techniques for lowering the risk of liver disease and assisting the liver in ridding the body of toxins include: Limiting alcohol consumption: Excessive alcohol intake raises the risk of liver damage. Those who are alcoholics should get treatment.

- **Preventing the use of unneeded over-the-counter medicines:** Never exceed the prescribed amount, especially for medicines that might damage the liver, such as acetaminophen. Do not combine alcohol and over-the-counter medications.

- **Selecting trustworthy tattoo and piercing salons:** Look for a salon that sterilizes its equipment. Hepatitis C can be spread by unsafe body alterations.
- **Obtaining a Vaccination:** Before traveling abroad, a person should be inoculated against hepatitis A and B and have all necessary vaccines.
- **Safe sex practice:** This can minimize the chance of spreading liver-related diseases. People should also be checked for sexually transmitted diseases on a regular basis (STIs).
- **Keeping potentially hazardous substances at bay:** Wear a mask and keep the area properly ventilated when painting or applying insecticides.

Consume a liver-friendly diet.

This should come as no surprise, but your diet has a big impact on your liver's overall health.

To guarantee that your diet is a long-term benefit to your liver, consider the following:
- **Consume a variety of foods.** Whole grains, fruits and vegetables, lean protein, dairy, and healthy fats are all good choices. Grapefruit, blueberries, almonds, and fatty fish are all known to have liver-friendly properties.
- **Consume an adequate amount of fiber.** Fiber is necessary for your liver to operate properly. Fruits and vegetables, as well as whole grains, are excellent sources of fiber to include in your diet.
- **Stay hydrated.** Drink plenty of water every day to maintain your liver in good health.
- **Consume less fatty, sugary, and salty foods.** Foods rich in fat, sugar, and salt can have a long-term impact on liver

function. Fried and quick meals might also harm your liver's health.

- **Drink coffee.** Coffee consumption has been linked to a decreased risk of liver illnesses such as cirrhosis and liver cancer. It works by inhibiting the buildup of fat and collagen, both of which contribute to liver damage.

Exercise regularly

Physical activity is beneficial to more than just your musculoskeletal and cardiovascular systems. It is also beneficial to your liver.

A 2018 study looked at the impact of exercise in non-alcoholic fatty liver disease (NAFLD), which is currently one of the most frequent liver disorders. The researchers came to the conclusion that both aerobic and resistance workouts aid in the prevention of fat accumulation in the liver. NAFLD is related to fat accumulation.

You don't have to run marathons to profit. You may begin exercising right now by going for a brisk walk, joining an online exercise class, or going for a bike ride.

3

How to Stop Smoking

Most smokers are aware that smoking is unhealthy for their health and dangerous to others around them. They know they should stop, but they also know it will be difficult. The majority of smokers have attempted to stop previously.

Why is it so difficult to quit?

Although we are all aware of the hazards of smoking, this does not make quitting any easier. Quitting smoking, whether you're a casual adolescent smoker or a pack-a-day smoker, may be tough.

Tobacco addiction is both physical and psychological. Cigarette nicotine produces a brief (and addictive) high. When you stop getting your nicotine fix on a regular basis, your body goes through physical withdrawal symptoms and cravings. Because nicotine has a "feel good" impact on the brain, you may turn to cigarettes as a quick and dependable method to improve your mood, alleviate stress, and unwind. Smoking can also be used to cope with sadness, anxiety, and boredom. Quitting entails learning new, better methods to deal with those sensations.

Smoking is entrenched as a regular routine as well. Smoking a cigarette with your morning coffee, at a break at work or school, or on your way home at the end of a long day may be an automatic response for you. Maybe your friends, family, or co-workers smoke, and it's become a part of how you interact with them.

To effectively stop smoking, you must address both the addiction and the habits and routines that go along with it. It is, nevertheless, conceivable. Even if they've tried and failed before, every smoker may conquer their addiction with the right help and stop plan.

Your personal STOP smoking plan

While some smokers succeed by quitting cold turkey, most individuals do better with a customized strategy to keep them on track. A good quit plan covers both the immediate issue of quitting smoking and the long-term challenge of avoiding relapse. It should also be customized to your individual requirements and smoking patterns.

Self-evaluation questions

Consider your smoking habits, as well as what circumstances in your life require the use of a cigarette and why. This can help you figure out which ideas, methods, or treatments will be the most beneficial to you.

Do you smoke a lot (at least a pack a day)? Or do you like to smoke in social situations? Is a basic nicotine patch enough? Do you have any activities, locations, or people in mind that you associate with smoking? Do you feel driven to smoke after every meal or whenever you go for a coffee break?

When you're anxious or sad, do you resort to smoking? Is there a link between your cigarette smoking and other addictions, such as alcohol or gambling?

START with START strategy when it comes to quitting smoking.

S = Set a deadline for quitting

Choose a date within the following two weeks to give yourself enough time to prepare without losing desire to stop. If you mostly smoke at work, stop on the weekend, so you have a few days to acclimatize.

T = Tell family, friends, and co-workers

Inform your friends and family of your plans to stop smoking, and let them know that you'll need their help and encouragement to succeed. Find a quit buddy who is also trying to stop smoking. You can assist one another in getting through difficult times.

A = Anticipate and prepare for the difficulties you'll encounter when quitting

The majority of people who re-start smoking do it within three months after quitting. You may help yourself get through by planning for frequent obstacles like nicotine withdrawal and cigarette cravings ahead of time.

R = Remove Cigarettes and other stuff like tobacco items from your house, vehicle, and workplace

Toss out all of your smokes, lighters, ashtrays, and matches. Wash your clothing and air out anything that has a smoky odor. Shampoo your automobile, steam your furniture, and clean your curtains and rugs.

T = Talk your doctor about obtaining assistance to stop smoking

Your doctor may prescribe medication to help you cope with withdrawal symptoms. If you are unable to visit a doctor, several products, including nicotine patches, lozenges, and gum, are available over the counter at your local drugstore.

Identify your smoking triggers

Identifying the things that make you want to smoke, such as specific circumstances, activities, feelings, and people is one of the finest things you can do to help yourself stop.

Maintain a cravings journal.

A craving notebook might assist you in identifying trends and triggers. Keep a smoking diary for a week or so before your stop date.

Keep track of the moments throughout the day when you feel the need to smoke:
- Could you tell me what time it was?
- How strong was the yearning (on a scale of 1 to 10)?
- What were you up to?
- With whom were you?
- How did you feel?
- How did you feel after you smoked?

Do you smoke to get rid of bad feelings?

Many of us smoke to cope with negative emotions, including stress, despair, loneliness, and worry. When you're having a terrible day, cigarettes might seem like your only buddy. However, as much as cigarettes give comfort, it is vital to realize that there are healthier and more efficient methods to deal with negative sensations. Exercising, meditating, relaxation techniques, or basic breathing exercises are examples of these.

For many individuals, finding other strategies to deal with uncomfortable feelings without turning to cigarettes is a crucial part of quitting smoking. Even if cigarettes are no longer a part of your life, the painful and unpleasant sentiments that drove you to smoke in the past will remain. So it's worth devoting some time to considering how you intend to deal with stressful circumstances and minor irritations that would ordinarily set you off.

Advice on how to avoid typical triggers

Alcohol: When they drink, many individuals smoke. Switch to non-alcoholic beverages or consume exclusively in locations where smoking is not permitted. Some alternatives include snacking on almonds, chewing on a cocktail stick, or sucking on a straw.

Other smokers: When friends, relatives, and co-workers smoke around you, quitting or avoiding relapse can be doubly tough. Talk about your decision to stop so that others know they won't be allowed to smoke with you in the car or at a coffee break. Find nonsmokers to have your breaks with at work, or find alternative activities to do, such as going for a walk.

End of a meal: For some smokers, finishing a meal means lighting up, and the idea of quitting might be scary. However, you may try substituting something different at that time after a meal, such as a piece of fruit, a nutritious dessert, a square of chocolate, or a stick of gum.

Coping with nicotine withdrawal symptoms

When you stop smoking, your body will most likely suffer a range of physical symptoms as it withdraws from nicotine.

Nicotine withdrawal often begins within an hour after the last smoke and peaks two to three days later. Withdrawal symptoms can last anywhere from a few days to many weeks and vary from person to person.

The following are some of the most frequent nicotine withdrawal symptoms:
- Cigarette cravings
- Irritability, irritation, or hostility
- Anxiety or anxiety
- Difficulty focusing

- Restlessness
- Increased hunger
- Headache
- Insomnia
- Tremors
- Increased coughing
- Fatigue
- Constipation or upset stomach
- Depression
- Reduced heart rate

As uncomfortable as these withdrawal symptoms are, keep in mind that they are only temporary. They will improve in a few weeks when the poisons are eliminated from your body.

Meanwhile, inform your friends and family that you will not be your regular self and beg for their understanding.

Manage cigarette cravings

While avoiding smoking triggers can help lessen your desire to smoke, you won't be able to completely eliminate cigarette cravings. Cravings, fortunately, don't last long—typically, 5 to 10 minutes. If you're tempted to smoke, tell yourself that the urge will pass and strive to resist. It is essential to plan ahead of time by developing ways to deal with cravings.

Distract yourself: Do the dishes, watch television, take a shower, or contact a buddy. It doesn't matter what you do as long as it takes your mind from smoking.

Remind yourself why you quit: Concentrate on your motivations for quitting, like the health benefits (reducing your risk of heart disease and lung cancer, for example), improved looks, money saved, and increased self-esteem.

Get out of a tempting situation: The need might be triggered by where you are or what you are doing. If this is the case, a change of location can make all the difference.

Reward yourself: Consolidate your successes. Give yourself a gift whenever you defeat a need to keep yourself motivated.

Managing cigarette urges in the present:
Look for an oral alternative — Keep alternative foods on hand to pop in your mouth when cravings strike. Mints, carrot or celery sticks, gum, or sunflower seeds are all healthy alternatives. Alternatively, take a sip via a drinking straw.

Keep your mind busy — Play an online game, read a book or magazine, listen to music, do a crossword or Sudoku problem, or read a book or magazine. Keep your hands busy - Tactile stimulation may be replaced by squeeze balls, pencils, or paper clips.
Brush your teeth — The sensation of having just brushed your teeth might help reduce cigarette cravings.

Drink water — Sip a big glass of water slowly. Staying hydrated not only helps the urge pass but also helps to reduce the symptoms of nicotine withdrawal. Light something else - Instead of smoking, burn a candle or some incense.

Get active — Take a stroll, do some jumping jacks or pushups, try some yoga stretches, or go for a run around the block.

Try to relax — Calm yourself down by taking a warm bath, meditating, reading a book, or performing deep breathing techniques. Go somewhere smoking is not permitted - For example, enter a public facility, store, mall, coffee shop, or movie theater.

How to avoid weight gain after quitting smoking

Because smoking suppresses appetite, gaining weight is a typical concern for many of us when we decide to quit smoking. You could even be using it as an excuse not to quit. While it is true that many smokers gain weight within six months of quitting, the rise is often small—about five pounds on average—and the initial gain diminishes with time. It's also crucial to realize that gaining a few pounds for a few months won't harm your heart as much as smoking does. However, gaining weight is NOT an unavoidable consequence of quitting smoking.

Because smoking dulls your sense of smell and taste, meals will frequently appear more attractive when you quit. You may also gain weight if you substitute smoking's oral satisfaction with unhealthy comfort foods. As a result, rather than mindless, emotional eating, it is critical to discover alternative, healthier methods to deal with undesirable sensations such as stress, worry, or boredom.

Nurture yourself: When you are worried, nervous, or sad, instead of reaching for smokes or food, find new techniques to comfort yourself rapidly. For example, listen to cheerful music, play with a pet, or enjoy a cup of hot tea.

Eat healthy, varied meals. Consume plenty of fruits and vegetables, as well as healthy fats. Avoid sugary foods, drinks, fried foods, and fast food.

Learn to eat with awareness. Emotional eating is almost always automatic and unthinking. It's simple to eat an ice cream tub while zoning out in front of the TV or gazing at your phone. However, avoiding distractions when eating allows you to focus on how much you're eating and tune into your body and how you're truly feeling. Are you still hungry or do you have another motive to eat?

Consume plenty of water. Drinking at least six to eight 8-ounce glasses of water each day will help you feel full and prevent you from eating when you aren't hungry. Water will also aid in the removal of toxins from your body.

Take a stroll. It will not only help you burn calories and keep the weight off, but it will also help you deal with the stress and anguish that comes with quitting smoking.

Snack on meals that are guilt-free. Sugar-free gum, carrot and celery sticks, sliced bell peppers, and jicama are all healthy alternatives.

Medication and therapy to help you quit

There are several techniques that have effectively assisted people in quitting smoking. While the first approach you attempt may be effective, it is more likely that you will need to try a number of other methods or a mix of therapies to find the ones that work best for you.

Medications

Smoking cessation medicines can lessen cravings and alleviate withdrawal symptoms. They are most successful when taken in conjunction with a thorough quit smoking program overseen by your doctor. Consult your doctor about your alternatives and if an anti-smoking drug is appropriate for you. The following are U.S. Food and Drug Administration (FDA) approved alternatives in the United States.

Nicotine replacement therapy

Nicotine replacement treatment is substituting nicotine substitutes such as nicotine gum, patch, lozenge, inhaler, or nasal spray for cigarettes. It alleviates certain withdrawal symptoms by providing tiny and consistent amounts of nicotine into your body without the tars and toxic chemicals present in cigarettes. This form of treatment allows you to focus on overcoming your psychological addiction while also making it simpler to acquire new behaviors and coping abilities.

Non-nicotine medication

These drugs assist you in quitting smoking by decreasing cravings and withdrawal symptoms without the usage of nicotine. Bupropion (Zyban) and varenicline (Chantix, Champix) are only indicated for short-term usage.

Alternative therapies

There are numerous alternatives to nicotine replacement treatment, vaping, or prescription medicines for quitting smoking.

These are some examples:

Hypnosis - This is a popular choice that has helped many smokers who are trying to stop. Forget what you've seen from stage hypnotists; hypnosis works by putting you in a deeply relaxed state where you're susceptible to ideas that reinforce your commitment to quitting smoking while increasing your negative sentiments about cigarettes.

Acupuncture - Acupuncture, one of the oldest known medical treatments, is thought to operate by causing the release of endorphins (natural pain relievers) that allow the body to relax. Acupuncture can assist in managing smoking withdrawal symptoms as a smoking cessation therapy.

Behavioral Therapy - Nicotine addiction is linked to smoking's regular actions or routines. Behavior therapy focuses on developing new coping strategies and changing bad habits.

Motivational Therapies — Self-improvement Books and websites can provide a variety of methods for motivating yourself to quit smoking. Calculating monetary savings is a well-known example. Some people have found an incentive to quit just by estimating how much money they will save. It may be enough to cover the cost of summer vacation.

Smokeless tobacco or spit tobacco is NOT a healthy substitute for smoking. Smokeless tobacco, often known as spit or chewing tobacco, is not a healthy substitute for smoking cigarettes. It includes nicotine, the same addictive substance found in cigarettes. In fact, the quantity of nicotine absorbed through smokeless tobacco can be three to four times that of a cigarette.

What should you do if you slip or relapse?

Most individuals try to quit smoking numerous times before they succeed, so don't be too hard on yourself if you slip up and smoke a cigarette. Instead, by learning from your error, you may convert your relapse into a rebound. Analyze what happened just before you started smoking again, discover the triggers or difficult places you encountered, and devise a fresh quit-smoking strategy that avoids them.

It is also critical to distinguish between a slip and a relapse. If you reintroduce smoking, it does not preclude you from resuming your abstinence.

You may either learn from your slip and use it to motivate you to do more in the future, or you can use it as an excuse to continue smoking. The choice, though, is completely yours. A slip does not have to result in a complete relapse.

If you make a mistake, you are not a failure. It doesn't mean you can't give up for good. Don't allow a slip to turn into a mudslide. Throw the remainder of the pack away. It is critical to returning to a nonsmoking lifestyle as soon as feasible.

Look back at your quit log and be proud of the time you spent without smoking. Find the cause. What prompted you to start smoking again? Determine how you will handle the situation the next time it arises.

Learn from your mistakes. What has been the most beneficial? So, what didn't work? Are you using medication to help you quit smoking? If you begin smoking again, contact your doctor. Some medications cannot be used if you are also smoking.

Aiding a loved one to quit smoking

It is critical to realize that you cannot force a friend or loved one to quit smoking; the decision must be theirs. However, if they do decide to stop smoking, you may give support and encouragement while also attempting to alleviate the stress of quitting. Investigate the many treatment alternatives available and discuss them with the smoker; however, never preach or judge. You may also assist a smoker in overcoming cravings by engaging in other activities with them and keeping smoking alternatives available, like gum.

Don't make a loved one feel bad if they stumble or relapse. Congratulate them on their cigarette-free period and urge them to try again. Your aid can make all the difference in helping your loved one quit smoking for good.

Assisting an Adolescent in quitting smoking

Most smokers begin smoking around the age of 11, and many are hooked by the age of 14. In recent years, the usage of e-cigarettes (vaping) has also increased rapidly. While the health consequences of vaping are not completely understood, the FDA advises that it is not safe for teenagers, and we do know that kids who vape are more likely to start smoking cigarettes. This might be concerning for parents, but it is crucial to recognize the specific obstacles and peer pressure that teenagers experience while trying to quit smoking (or vaping). While the choice to quit smoking must be made by the young smoker, there are several ways you may assist.

Tips for Parents of Smoking or Vaping Adolescents

Determine why your kid is smoking or vaping; they may want to be accepted by their classmates or seek your attention. Rather than issuing threats or ultimatums, discuss what adjustments may be done in their lives to assist them in quitting smoking.

If your child agrees to stop, be patient and supportive of their efforts.

Set a positive example by refusing to smoke. Smoking parents are more likely to have smoking children. Determine why your kid is smoking or vaping; they may want to be accepted by their classmates or seek your attention. Rather than issuing threats or ultimatums, discuss what adjustments may be done in their lives to assist them in quitting smoking.

If your child agrees to stop, be patient and supportive of their efforts. Set a positive example by refusing to smoke. Smoking parents are more likely to have smoking children.

4

Dr. Sebi's Hair Loss Treatment

Many men and women are concerned about hair loss. There are several causes of hair loss, ranging from genetics and vitamin deficiencies to hormonal shifts. Medical conditions such as thyroid illness may also cause hair loss or thinning.

There is no magic pill for increasing hair, but studies have shown that some herbs can help reduce hair loss or encourage new growth. It should be noted, however, that much of the study has been conducted on animals. More study is required in people to prove their effectiveness.

Continue reading to find out how doctor Sebi's herbal medicines might help you grow your hair faster. Before incorporating herbs into your daily regimen, consult with your doctor, especially if your hair loss is caused by a medical issue.

Treatment of hair loss in Dr. Sebi's way

Dr. Sebi used charged alkaline meals, which offer the key vitamins, minerals, and amino acids required for hair development. Dr. Sebi's selection of alkaline herbs aids in the nourishment of the hair and scalp. The herbs promote hair development, battle male baldness, prevent hair thinning, and strengthen and nourish existing hair to avoid additional hair loss.

The Medicinal Constituents Found in Each Herb That Makes It Effective:
- Coconut oil

- Batana oil
- Olive oil
- French vanilla
- Drops Lavender

Coconut oil

Coconut oil is an edible oil made from the flesh of mature coconuts harvested from the coconut palm. The nut's oil is used to create medication. Virgin coconut oil is a term used to describe some coconut oil products. The phrase has evolved to indicate that the oil is unprocessed in general. Virgin coconut oil, for example, is not generally bleached, deodorized, or refined. Coconut oil has 87g of saturated fat, 1.8g of polyunsaturated fat, and 6g of monounsaturated fat. Coconut oil helps to reduce protein loss and easily penetrates the hair shaft for conditioning. It stimulates hair development and makes it thicker and longer. Furthermore, coconut oil helps to seal in moisture while also providing a pleasant glow and gloss. When applying coconut oil, damaged hair is resurrected.

Batana oil

Batana oil is derived from the nut of the palm tree, which grows naturally in the tropical rainforests of Central and South America. This oil is quite helpful for promoting long hair growth. The residents of Honduras, where Doctor Sebi lived, refer to it as a miracle oil. People who use this oil have gorgeous, long, and glossy hair. Tocopherols, Omega-6 linoleic acid, carotenoids, phytosterols, and other active components are included in the oil. The following functions are aided by banana oil: It aids in the restoration and nourishment of damaged hair. It aids in the regrowth of dry hair. It aids in the curling of the hair. It aids in the thickening of the hair. It contributes to the gloss of the hair. It keeps gray hair at bay. It fortifies the hair. It promotes hair growth.

Olive oil

Olive oil is a kind of lipid-derived from the fruit of the olive tree. This oil includes the following active components, which make it helpful against hair loss, hair damage, and hair infections, as well as promoting hair growth: K-vitamin. Fatty acids are essential fatty acids. The antioxidant vitamin E. Components that reduce inflammation.

Olive oil offers the following hair benefits:

It gets rid of dandruff. It encourages hair growth. It softens the hair. It aids in the alleviation of scalp inflammation. It causes hair to grow longer. It hydrates the hair.

French vanilla

The vanilla plant is a herbaceous climbing vine that grows best when supported by a tree or pole. Vanilla beans are used to make this oil. When used as an essential oil, vanilla helps strengthen the hair and increase blood flow to the scalp, encouraging hair growth. This oil makes your hair smooth, soft, and manageable while preventing breaking. Furthermore, French vanilla promotes hair development, making hair smoother, fuller, and shinier while also imparting an enticing aroma.

Lavender oil

Lavender oil has the following effects on your hair: It aids in the treatment of scalp inflammatory conditions. It helps to prevent lice as well as destroys them. Lavender oil is used to treat bacterial and fungal diseases of the scalp. Lavender aids in the prevention of scalp irritation. Lavender aids in the treatment of dandruff. Lavender aids in the growth of new hair.

The General Preparation of Dr. Sebi Hair Growth Herbal Medicines Herbal Items:

- 40 Drops of Coconut oil.
- 20 Drop of Batana oil.
- 20 Drops of Olive oil.
- 10 Drops of French vanilla.
- 10 Drops of Lavender.

Hair Growth Oil Blend Preparation

1. Obtain a sample bottle with a dispensing tube.
2. Fill the sample vial with the required number of drops of the herbal component.
3. Shake the mixture thoroughly before applying it to your hair.

Boiling Method for Hair Growth Soap Preparation

1. Get 100g of your favorite bathing solid soaps (Natural Soap) rather than Skin Bleaching, Toning, or Antiseptic Soap.
2. Make a bow out of the soap.
3. Fill a cooking pot with 30-50ml of water.
4. Pour the thinly cut soaps into the water-filled saucepan.
5. Place the saucepan on a heating device/medium, heat, and stir until the soap is completely melted.
6. Remove from the heat source and stir in 1-2 teaspoons of the above oil blend from the sample container.
7. Stir the oil into the melted soap, then pour it all into a small container to harden.
8. Use soap to wash your hair in the morning and at night.
9. After each bath, the hair growth mixes oil to your hair to feed and strengthen it.

Cold Method

1. Obtain 100g of your preferred bathing solid soaps.
2. Slice the soap into a bow.
3. In order to prepare the cold technique, soak the thinly sliced soap in Coconut water.
4. Cover the bowl with coconut water that has been leveled with sliced soap.
5. Allow 48 hours for the soap to soften fully and be ready to form a paste when stirred or pounding.
6. Pound it with a pestle and mortar until smooth.
7. Alternatively, use a stirrer to fully mix the soap until it is thoroughly combined.
8. Place it in a jar and cover it with a lid.
9. Use it to wash your hair in the morning and at night, and then use the Hair Growth Blend Oil generously to nourish the hair.

Preparation of Cream:

Hair Cream

1. Combine 2–4 teaspoons of Hair Growth Blend Oil with 25–50ml of your preferred Hair Cream.
2. If you have waxy hair cream.
3. Place the bottom of the petroleum waxy jelly bottle in a basin of boiling water for 10-15 minutes to melt the waxy hair cream.
4. Pour in the appropriate amount of the hair growth oil combination and carefully mix it in.
5. Remove it from the boiling water and set it aside to cool.
6. Use it to massage your hair after a wash in the morning and evening.
7. However, ladies must apply it to their hair twice daily.

Hair Lotion

1. To 25ml–50ml Hair Cream Lotion, add 2–4 tablespoons of Hair Growth Oil Blend.
2. Shake the tube vigorously to obtain an even mixing.
3. Rub it through your hair in the morning and evening. Female Hair Washing Schedule After washing your hair with Shampoo and Conditioner, apply the above Hair Growth Oil Blend straight to your hair and repeat the process for the following three days before continuing with the hair cream mixture (it is optional). You may continue to use the Hair Growth Oil Blend to promote quick and healthy hair growth.

Doctor Sebi's Other Herbs for Hair Growth Other significant herbs that are beneficial for hair growth and hair loss are as follows. Those herbs are edible and may be used to supplement your diet by adding ¼ teaspoon of powder.

These herbs are as follows:
- Marshmallow
- Watercress
- Nettle
- Thyme
- Flaxseed

5

Dr. Sebi Treatment for Heart Disease

The Dr. Sebi diet, commonly known as the Dr. Sebi alkaline diet, is a plant-based diet created by Dr. Sebi. It is said to renew your cells by removing harmful waste from your blood by alkalinizing it.

The diet consists of a limited number of permitted items as well as several supplements. This diet is based on the African Bio-Mineral Balance hypothesis and was created by self-taught herbalist Alfredo Darrington Bowman, often known as Dr. Sebi. Dr. Sebi, despite his name, was not a medical doctor or a Ph.D. holder.

He created this diet for everyone who wants to treat or prevent disease organically and enhance their general health without relying on conventional Western medicine.

Disease, according to Dr. Sebi, is caused by a buildup of mucus in a certain location of your body. For example, pneumonia is caused by a buildup of mucus in the lungs, but diabetes is caused by an excess of mucus in the pancreas.

He claims that illnesses cannot live in an alkaline environment and that they begin to manifest themselves when your body gets too acidic. He promises to restore your body's natural alkaline condition and cleanse your sick body by closely adhering to his diet and utilizing his unique, expensive supplements.

Our entire health is greatly influenced by the food we eat. There are several advantages to eating a more alkaline-based diet, including improved cardiovascular health, decreased blood pressure, and disease prevention.

The nine alkaline foods listed below can be added to the diet to help reduce blood pressure:

1. **Watermelon**
    Magnesium and potassium, both of which may be found in abundance in watermelon, can help to decrease blood pressure. Potassium works as a vasodilator, dilating blood vessels and assisting in the release of tension from veins and arteries. This increases blood flow and relieves stress on the cardiovascular system. Watermelon contains carotenoids as well. Organic pigments in the colors orange, red, and yellow give fruits and vegetables like maize, pumpkins, tomatoes, and carrots their distinctive hue. Carotenoids keep the walls of the arteries and veins from hardening, which lowers blood pressure.

2. **Plum Tomatoes**
    Eating one plum tomato per day lowers the risk of high blood pressure. This is mostly due to plum tomatoes' high potassium content, which lowers blood vessel stress. This improves circulation and reduces the pressure and stress on the heart.

3. **Walnuts**
    Consuming walnuts has been proven in studies to lower bad cholesterol levels while increasing good cholesterol levels. Eating around 25 grams of walnuts per day can supply approximately 90 percent of the required daily quantity of essential fatty acids. As a result, the chances of developing high blood pressure and heart disease are lowered.

4. Rye

Rye is regarded as a heart-healthy food. This is because it includes magnesium, which aids in heart health and blood pressure management. It also includes a lot of soluble fiber, which can help lower cholesterol. Rye is suggested for daily consumption since it includes a variety of vital nutrients that the body requires, as well as high fiber and mineral content.

5. Dandelion Greens

Urination is one of the most effective blood pressure-lowering methods, and most contemporary blood pressure medicines are based on this fact. Dandelion juice is diuretic by nature, which means it enhances both urine quality and frequency. As a result, it aids in the reduction of blood pressure.

6. Strawberries

Strawberries are also rich in potassium and magnesium, two minerals that may help lower blood pressure produced by inorganic sodium and other causes. Strawberries also lessen the stiffness of blood vessel walls, which lowers blood pressure.

7. Burdock Tea

Burdock tea has been shown to help reduce blood pressure. However, this is not commonly known. Burdock has a high potassium content, which relaxes the veins and arteries and reduces stress in the cardiovascular system. As a result, it aids in the prevention of heart attacks, strokes, and atherosclerosis, a condition in which plaque builds up inside the arteries.

8. Prickly Pears

Prickly pears are another heart-healthy dietary option. They contain a lot of potassium and help to decrease blood pressure by relaxing the blood vessels and reducing stress on the cardiovascular system.

9. Tomatillos

Tomatillos have a high potassium-to-sodium ratio, which can help lower blood pressure. Potassium improves oxygenation and circulation in the body, relaxes blood vessels, and lowers cardiovascular system pressure.

High blood pressure may create significant stress in the body, as well as the release of cortisol and other stress hormones. These, in turn, can be hazardous to one's health. Including these alkaline foods in your regular diet will help you retain excellent health and lower your blood pressure.

Conclusion

Dr. Sebi thought that mucus and acidity were the root causes of illness. He believed that consuming some foods and avoiding others might cleanse the body, resulting in an alkaline condition that could minimize illness risk and consequences.

Dr. Sebi's technique is very intriguing, concentrating on natural, alkaline, plant-based meals and herbs while avoiding acidic, hybrid foods that might harm the cell. You may avoid mucus buildup, which can contribute to illness development, by adopting Alfredo Bowman's (aka Dr. Sebi) method.

Dr. Sebi is the Honduran founder of the USHA Treatment Village, which not only offers to heal but also educates people on how to live an alkaline lifestyle. Because they were educated to believe in the medication method to treat patients, medical professionals sometimes feel that the Dr. Sebi herbal approach to cure sickness is useless.

Bowman is an inspiration to many people and a great herbalist since he developed a technique to treat life-threatening ailments that were previously thought to be incurable. He has been a herbalist for over 40 years and claims to be able to treat patients suffering from AIDS, asthma, cancer, diabetes, eczema, epilepsy, fibroids, heart disease, high blood pressure, inflammation, lupus, multiple sclerosis, and sickle cell disease, among other things.